STOUSH

STYLE SECRETS

10 Tips to Develop
Your Personal and
Professional Image!

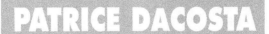

PATRICE DACOSTA

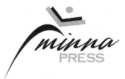

minna
PRESS

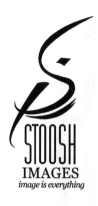

IMAGES
image is everything

Copyright © 2015 Patrice DaCosta
All Rights Reserved. No part of this publication
may be reproduced, stored in a retrieval system or
transmitted in any form or by any means, electronic,
mechanical, photocopying, recording or otherwise
without the permission of author or publisher.

Disclaimer: Some names and identifying details have
been changed to protect the privacy of individuals

A catalogue record of this book is available from the
National Library of Jamaica

ISBN: 978-976-95693-8-6

Executive Editor: Lena Joy Rose
Proofreader: Kiki Kimoto
Book design: Mark Weinberger
Illustrator: Damian Shaw

Published in Kingston, Jamaica by
Minna Press: www.minnapress.com
Ordering Information:
Quantity (Bulk) Sales: Special discounts are available
on quantity (bulk) purchases by corporations,
associations, and others. For details, contact the
publisher: sales@minnapress.com

DEDICATION

This book is dedicated to my mother,
Linnette DaCosta, for being my rock
and for those in my life
who have always had the confidence in what I do.

To my clients and friends
within the Caribbean region
(especially, Barbados, Trinidad, Jamaica)
who have been a consistent source of support
throughout the years.

ACKNOWLEDGEMENT

I have to say thank you Lord for granting me the opportunity to live my dreams, knowing I'm living on purpose. There are so many people I would like to say thanks to for being supportive over the years.

My clients, thanks for trusting me with your image, allowing me into your homes and respecting my opinions. You make what I do fulfilling. For all the stories, laughter, and tears shared, I thank you.

Special thanks to four individuals who have been my rock over the years. I could always share my thoughts and my fears, get encouragement and have them challenge me to reach greater heights: (i) My mentor, Jerry Blenman; (ii) My mom, Linnette DaCosta, this is the woman who had my back from inception; (iii) My aunt, Lena Rose, who has been a part of Stoosh, allowing me to believe that all things are possible even during the down times. (iv) Also, to my wonderful husband, Keston Fernandez, for his continuous support.

For all my family and friends, you know who you are, thank you for being a part of my life.

Cheers to lots more Stooshing!

CONTENTS

CONTENTS

PREFACE

Realize that you are judged by your appearance, even before your talent is noticed. As a result, you will become more aware of your appearance.

People react to you based on what they see.

I have had this realization all my life – the impact of appearance. In fact, my love for fashion and personal development started from the days of attending Westwood High School, an elite all-girls school I attended in the hills of Trelawny, Jamaica.

Flashback to the years of 1998-1990, at the beginning of high school I knew in my heart I loved fashion and grooming. I would coordinate colours, and invariably, I would get the response:

> *"I wouldn't think of that" or "how lovely, very elegant"*
> *or "how stoosh."*

Friends would choose me to accompany them on their clothes shopping trips. I began to hone my interest in the field by reading fashion magazines and speaking to experienced people in the fashion industry as well as attending fashion shows. I would even be asked to model at local events or coordinate fashion shows. So since I was a teenager, I recognized the importance of portraying a confident and well groomed image. I would see the difference in people's reaction to each other based on their appearance. This is somewhat unfortunate but it is reality.

I recall day dreaming about visiting Paris, boutique shopping and sitting in the front seat at a major designer runway show. Even though I have not yet visited Paris, I had the opportunity to attend a Diane von Fürstenberg show at fashion week in New York. Oh what a joy that was!

It is so fulfilling and worthwhile to me when I see my clients move from one level to the next in their self-enhancement. The remarks and questions that I would also get from strangers boosted and confirmed that I was doing something right. The simple techniques I used to create a stylish look became easier.

I believe no experience in life is wasted. After spending over 15 years in the travel industry, I know without a doubt that my heart belongs in the fashion/image industry. During that time, I travelled throughout the Caribbean immersing myself in the mores and norms of the various islands. This experience would prove to become the stepping stone for launching my fashion business.

Today, after years in the fashion business, the next step on my journey is to condense all my knowledge and experience into an easy reference book. My intention in writing this book is to create a style guide, to help develop your unique personal and professional image so you can step out with confidence!

Yours in style

Patrice

Patrice DaCosta

INTRODUCTION

*"...**STOOSH** IS STYLISH,
SOPHISTICATED
AND SUCCESSFUL."*—PATRICE DACOSTA

In 2005, Stoosh Images was born. Stoosh, a Jamaican word, can encompass a wide range of meanings from being self-aware, elegant and confident to being very stylish and unique. For me, Stoosh is stylish, sophisticated and successful.

As I meet many people in my path, I am amazed at the low levels of self-confidence that abound. This book, *Stoosh Style Secrets,* covers various aspect of professional development by giving tips, sharing my knowledge and helping to build self-confidence.

I believe this book will assist you in loving and appreciating your assets and liabilities. After reading this book you will realize that being stylish, sophisticated and appropriate is much easier than you can imagine. You will also be motivated to be the best you can.

The challenges shared by many include:

- Mixing a colour palette—what shade is complimentary to different skin tones or how to combine colours
- What to wear that is age appropriate
- How to accessorize
- Major issues with developing an appropriate business casual wardrobe
- Dealing with body challenges:
  My arms are big; I hate my knees; my stomach is

bulging; my breasts are too small, or too large; thighs and butt too fat; feet are big; neck is short; shoulders too broad…the list goes on and on

Read on and learn how to highlight your assets and camouflage your liabilities.

As I introduce this book, I encourage you to accept who you are and where you are right now—but don't be afraid to reach for the stars, for the sky's the limit when you become Stoosh!

Because you deserve to be.

Chapter One

ESTABLISH THE STOOSH POWER MINDSET

"A GIRL SHOULD BE TWO THINGS: CLASSY AND FABULOUS"—COCO CHANEL

The Stoosh mindset is realizing that each person possesses the potential to be more than they are right this very minute. Personal development should be a daily/ongoing aspect of life. I often share with my clients that if there is no desire to grow, to develop in a positive way, to make changes, to try new ideas then life becomes limiting and stagnant.

The ABC of Image

Being Stoosh is not only dealing with the outward appearance but your behavior and communication also known as the "ABC of image"—Appearance, Behavior and Communication. When these three areas are on the same level you radiate such confidence and energy that your very presence makes a unique statement wherever you go.

Do you know your appearance is your visual resume?

Contrary to what some might believe, your attire speaks before you have the chance to utter your first word. You speak before opening your mouth.

First impressions are very easy to form but hard to undo. Do you know 67% of first impressions are usually correct? We know it takes one or two seconds to make a first impression.

What impression are you making on a daily basis?

80% ATTENTION OF YOUR AUDIENCE IS DRAWN TO HOW YOU PRESENT YOURSELF, 20% TOWARDS YOUR MESSAGE.

A Stoosh mindset is not dependent on body size. You dress for the size you are not the size you want to be. I enjoy consulting with full-figured ladies, especially the ones who realize that looking stylish and successful is not only for thinner women. Success comes in every shape, size and form. The key is knowing what are your assets and liabilities (we will discuss further in the book). Dress to represent you now and what best suits you now.

Opportunity does not always lend itself to spending time getting to know you, so ensure your split second impression is showing your highest potential. This is not always easy but aim to put your best forward at all times. Research suggests that our clothes influence others and change our own behavior as well.

What if I told you that having a Stoosh mindset builds your credibility and makes it easier to influence others? Life in general is easier as you deal with others. Research by Dr. Mehrabian, of UCLA, found our credibility is based on three factors:

1. Verbal – what you say
2. Vocal – how you say it
3. Visual – your facial expressions and your image

Can you guess which had the highest percentage?

The result is 55% visual.

Consequently, taking care of how you look, what comes out of your mouth and being mindful of your behavior can bring you opportunities and success. For example, I have had the opportunity to be in mansions, to speak with prime ministers and ministers of government, diplomats, and high net worth individuals. Can you imagine, if these opportunities were presented to me and I did not have the confidence or the appropriate mindset to seize the moment? Or, if I allowed them to pass me by? This state of being did not happen overnight but by making a conscious decision and a constant effort to renew my mindset.

With daily effort, there is no doubt that eventually your confidence will rise, and the best part is, it will soon become apparent to you and everyone around you. Your creativity and uniqueness begin to flow as you tap into your potential. Your potential is to be maximized not minimized. Taking care of your mental and physical being gives you an advantage. If you can take care of you, spend the extra time to ensure that you are looking professional and appropriate, the universe will reward you. What you put out you get back.

Having a Stoosh mindset, shows you are capable/classy/ready for opportunities. Some elements of being Stoosh are knowing your body type, your lifestyle, what are your complimentary colours, what to wear when, what is age appropriate, what to say and not to say. It is a beautiful thing to have such a mindset. My clients can confirm this as many have seen their lives spiral upwards, in various areas, soon after they begin living out this mindset. I get comments such as:

> *"My thinking is different, my self-confidence has improved, my marriage or relationship is renewed, and I spend less as I am more focused."*

Being Stoosh not only affects your professional but also your personal life. How you relate to your peers, the opposite sex, your spouse and others will be impacted.

PEOPLE SPEAK TO YOU BASED ON WHAT THEY SEE. WHEN YOU RESPECT YOURSELF TO TAKE CARE OF YOU, OTHERS WILL RESPECT YOU.

You can command respect without asking for it, by consistently displaying a good image (ABC).

It is interesting that many mothers confess to losing themselves and their sense of style after having a child.

HAVING A CHILD IS NOT AN EXCUSE FOR LOOKING TEN YEARS OLDER OR LOOKING LIKE YOU NO LONGER CARE ABOUT YOURSELF.

Remember that your child needs a role model and as they get older they will want to emulate you. If there is nothing to emulate they often look elsewhere and sometimes that's not the best choice.

Balance

Achieving balance is the Stoosh way and often will result in a better lifestyle for you. So many husbands have thanked me for building their spouse's self-confidence and improving their intimate relations. There is a chain reaction to having such a mindset. It affects every area in your life.

Signature Style

Establishing such a mindset propels you to build your "signature style" and fashion style. What is your signature?

Ask yourself the question:

What do I wear a lot? Is it unique accessories, a certain type of pocket book, high or flat shoes, dresses versus pants, scarves, brooches, a certain hairstyle, or specific lipstick?

Think about it and identify your signature style as it helps you to form your unique look and assist you in evaluating the areas that need to be improved. Sometimes we are stuck in a rut for years before we realize that we can make adjustments.

Here are seven fashion styles that can help you identify your style. Which one or two are you?

1. Alluring
2. Feminine
3. Traditional/classic
4. Dramatic
5. Sporty
6. Creative
7. Elegant

Knowing yourself, is a big part of being Stoosh. This will prevent you from seeing outfits in the store and becoming confused by what suits your style and the image you want to reflect to the world.

Your image is your valuable "you" asset. Why not nourish and make it a priority when the outcomes are so positive? It is very easy to make excuses: "I can't do this, I'm scared, I don't know", we go on and on. Remember one thing:

Do not hinder yourself. Stop settling for less when you deserve more.

What do you deserve?

- You deserve to have a positive mindset
- You deserve to have a wardrobe that works for you
- You deserve to be successful and become even more successful
- You deserve to be your best

WHATEVER YOUR POSITION OR STATUS IN LIFE THERE IS ALWAYS MORE ROOM TO GROW AND GLOW.

Your image will take you as high as you want to go.
How high do you want to go?

Five How to be Stoosh Tips

1. Identify where you are in your life and where you want to go. Visual (*see yourself*). Affirm (*there is so much power in our words*) and Act (what should I do, what steps should I take).

2. Surround yourself with people who have the same mindset. As the old adage goes: "You can't soar like an eagle when you hang out with turkeys". Or another one that says: "If you hang with eagles you will begin to soar, if you lay with pigs you begin to think and act like them". So, hang around your tigers, the people who strengthen, encourage and challenge you to be your best.

3. Realise you are just as important as your spouse, your children, your parents. Make the effort to take care of self. Your kids need you as a positive role model.

4. Acknowledge your negative traits but aim to correct them and be the best you. Opportunity doesn't always come knocking. Ensure when it comes you open the door and do not block your growth. Refrain from saying "this is just me or this is how I am". You are a living, breathing entity, so development and change is a given.

5. Be mindful of your attitude and etiquette especially when you are speaking with others. Let people enjoy having you in their space. Acknowledge and treat people well. Remember what you give out comes right back.

Chapter Two

FINDING YOUR FLATTERING COLOURS

"I FOUND I COULD SAY THINGS
WITH COLOUR AND SHAPES
THAT I COULDN'T SAY ANY OTHER WAY—
THINGS I HAD NO WORDS FOR."
—GEORGIA O'KEEFFE

Women Radiate Confidence with Colour

Colour is one of my favourite topics, as it is often overlooked by many, yet so important. Colour imparts so much energy both good and bad. It's not the colour but the shade that makes all the difference in whether we radiate a glow or we look ten years older.

The right colour is your most important accessory, do not leave home without it.

Do you know that wearing your right colours in the right fabrics can hide your flaws? The key is to create the "eye-up principle" this is when the focus is on your face or neckline which detracts from the flaws.

For example, a bulging stomach/thick thighs/thin legs (these are some of the complaints I hear from my clients). When you wear colours that are stunning or colours that make a statement—a striking earring, necklace, jacket or blouse will create visual interest. Wearing the right colours near your face reflect light upwards, enhancing your appearance.

" *When Patrice made me aware of the colours that are right for me, it was a eureka moment! These colours reflect beauty and shades that enhance my personality, sense of style and confidence. They positively impacted my mood, energy and posture and made a significant and long-lasting impression, which I believe is important to share with others.*

The result is that I am a recipient of many an admiring glance, compliments and queries about my chic and colourful sense of style.

I now shop with an awareness and self-assurance that I know exactly what colours are best suited for my complexion and personality. The experience has also saved me much time, money and agony in the process.

My wish is that every woman (and man) would have the opportunity to experience such verve and excitement in exploring what colours are best suited for their style, complexion and personality. "

—MARCELLINE C

KNOWING YOUR BEST COLOURS CAN PROJECT SELF-CONFIDENCE AND A POSITIVE SELF-IMAGE.

The Right Fabrics in the Right Colours

Along with the right colours, your choice of fabrics is another critical element in radiating confidence. Your body type and the level of professionalism you want to display will be a deciding factor. For example, flimsy fabric on a full figured individual is not the ideal choice as the extra curves will be pronounced. Also, the placement of details or patterns on the fabric will add or reduce volume on your body.

Quick Tip

IF THE FABRIC DOESN'T CONTAIN ELASTANE OR SPANDEX, PURCHASE A SIZE UP, HOWEVER IF THE FABRIC HAS 3% OR MORE SPANDEX, PURCHASE ONE SIZE SMALLER.

Your Wardrobe Colours

Many people have a poor relationship with their wardrobe, not realizing that styles, colours and looks depict who they are on an external level. As I review many peoples' wardrobes, it saddens me when the colours of the clothing do not reflect the owner's personality. I do notice that people often gravitate to colours mainly because it is safe, or it's the trend, not necessarily what is right for the person.

Typically, the darker the colour the thinner you will look; the brighter the colour the bigger you appear. Dark colours do not have to be black—which is often the belief. Great dark colour options include burgundy, navy, charcoal grey, chocolate brown, hunter and teal greens.

Owning a wardrobe with the right shades that enhance you will make all the difference in your confidence and creativity. Yes creativity. Think about when you are wearing a colour that you know looks good on you or when you get a lot of compliments, how do you feel? I'm sure good, positive, confident, and creative.

Your Skin Colour Undertone

We have different skin colour undertones which affect how colours relate to us. The cool undertone has more blue, pink, olive greens while the warm undertone has more yellow, orange. Do you know your undertone? If not, there's no better time than the present to find out.

Please do not ignore what the right colours can do for you. Many of my clients before getting their colours analyzed would wear certain colours for years, they would often say this is what they know, or it's safe. They are not aware whether these safe shades are the appropriate ones for them.

Black is not for everyone (yes I said it). It is a common belief that black is a must. Wrong! Yes black is a great neutral and helps decrease volume. As with any other neutrals or colour, if not worn correctly or the fit is poor, black can be inappropriate. However, your undertone is critical. Black on some people can be harsh, aging and dull.

Mixing and Blending

Neutrals are great mixers if you're not sure how to combine colours. Neutrals consist of black, brown, white, navy, gray and khaki. These can be mixed with any colour. Adding colour to your neutral will add oomph and pizzazz. Wearing a detailed and sophisticated neutral is also very stoosh. I encourage you to avoid becoming stagnant and try something new. Enjoy and embrace colours (the right ones).

You deserve to glow, to be radiant, to look age appropriate, to enhance yourself as you mature, and to look royal. Yes that's what colour can do.

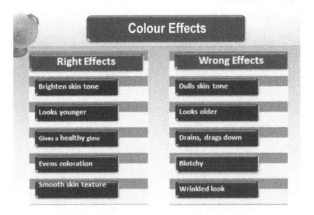

In the professional world, darker colours are perceived to be more formal, authoritative, bold, strong and sometimes masculine. Lighter colours are perceived to be less formal, warmer and sociable. The important thing is to have the right balance and not to always be looking the same way. How others see you can be dependent on the colours you wear. In certain industries such as legal and financial, darker colours may be appropriate. However, be reminded, you are not at work 24/7. When you can, add some colours (not just any, but the right ones) to your outfit.

Monochromatic shades and tints are of the same hue. This gives the illusion of length. High contrast such as black and white can shorten and cut you in half and thought must be taken when wearing this very popular combination.

Examples of monochromatic colours are:

- Beige/brown
- Royal blue/light blue
- Lavender/purple

"*Before my colour consultation with image consultant Patrice, I wore any colour and worse yet, matched all my accessories with every outfit. That was a drab look but I was only sensitized to it after receiving Patrice's expert advice when I learnt which colours worked best for my complexion and how to complement my colours instead of matching everything. With a shift in mindset on complementing accessories with my colour code, I added a boost to my dressing. My outfits are more stylish reflecting Stoosh Images. I spend less money on accessories as I learnt how to coordinate and complement several outfits. My confidence level rose as my conscientious efforts became natural to wear the correct colours each time while being creative in doing so. Others are drawn to my outfits and compliment the changed look. Sticking to my right colours gives me a vibrant vigorous look and the noticeable change causes others to comment positively.*"

—FAY W

NB: Monochromatic doesn't have to be all plain colours, a print with similar shade can be used which would add interest.

Colour experts reveal ten universal colours that flatter nearly everyone:

- Soft white
- Bright burgundy
- Medium gray
- Medium turquoise
- Blue violet
- Watermelon red
- Medium violet
- Coral or warm pink

You can add zest to your appearance by wearing the right colours.

Real Men Wear Colour

What if I tell you real men do wear colour? A confident man wears his right colour with ease. He knows who he is without guessing about his masculinity. Men in general tend to stick with blue, white, gray, black, brown. It is often believed that pink and purple colours are not for men, but that is a myth.

It is a beautiful thing to see a man wearing his colours with confidence. Colour could be shown in shirts, ties, blazers and tie pins. The right colour on a man in no way takes away from his professional look.

Wearing colours automatically puts you in a good mood even when you're feeling low. The important factor with colour is the shade. As I mentioned earlier, the colour might not be right but finding the right shade is key.

Neutral colours are the same for men—as they are for women—black, gray, white, navy, brown and khaki. If you wear neutrals every day, everywhere, it's guaranteed you are going to begin to feel like a neutral person. A touch of colour adds that extra pizazz. If wearing neutrals is all you know, aim for neutrals with details and structure.

Men are allowed three combined patterns and colour at any one time. In other words, a patterned shirt can be paired with a patterned tie. The important thing is the blending in order to look well groomed.

Similar to females, men should wear complimentary colours close to the face to create harmony with facial features.

One stylish male stated:

"I often avoid a plain white shirt as getting a right shade of white is challenging to find".

Because of the limitations of men's wear i.e. shirt and pants/shorts, the focus should be on colour, details and structure.

Avoid wearing shocking bright solid colours to the office especially if your industry is conservative and highly service oriented. Inappropriate colours can be a distraction.

KNOWING YOUR APPROPRIATE SHADES WILL MAKE ALL THE DIFFERENCE.

Fellows, your colours and your colour combination can make all the difference in attracting female interest. Finding colours that complement you that do not clash is an important part of presenting yourself as a stylish man.

AS MUCH AS POSSIBLE, STAY WITHIN YOUR COLOUR PALETTE. AVOID SETTLING FOR UNFLATTERING COLOURS.

GETTING A COLOUR CONSULTATION IS A MUST, IT SAVES TIME, MONEY AND BUILDS YOUR SELF-CONFIDENCE.

Chapter Three

GETTING A WARDROBE THAT WORKS

"ANY ITEM IN YOUR WARDROBE SHOULD SATISFY ONE OF TWO CRITERIA: UTILITY AND JOY."—STACY LONDON

Essential Items You Must Have in Your Wardrobe

The essentials for your wardrobe should first be determined in segments. You want to ensure you have a holistic wardrobe that covers the following: casual, business casual, casually elegant, career, semi-formal, and formal.

I have discovered over the years, the weakest segments in most of my clients' wardrobe are casual and casually elegant. This weakness derives from accumulating basic and boring casual pieces. My experiences with clients have always been to upgrade their casual wear or to provide nice "in between" clothing that are transitional.

Before purchasing, it is best to have a few objectives in mind, such as:

- Purpose of the item?
- How many times will I wear it?
- How many places can I wear it to?
- Will it be a great addition to the current wardrobe?
- Is it of good quality?
- Am I buying just because I like it?

However, having a wardrobe filled with items just because it is on sale is not the most effective way of building a holistic wardrobe. When I am conducting a wardrobe audit, my clients do confess that certain items were purchased because they were on sale.

A cost per wear formula is highly recommended when purchasing:

$$\frac{\text{Cost of item}}{\text{Number of wears}} = \text{Cost per wearing}$$

$$\frac{\$200 \text{ suit}}{50 \text{ wears}} = \$4.00 \text{ per wear}$$

This formula is amazing especially if you are purchasing a high ticketed item and not sure how to proceed. Quality is often better than quantity.

Career
Black; navy; gray jacket
Black; navy; gray skirt; pants
White button shirt
Sheath dress
Cardigan
Neutral shoes
Pearl necklace and earring
Printed scarf
Brooches
Tote bag (travel/hold papers; computer gadgets)

Casual/Casually Elegant
Detailed flat shoes
Beaded/detailed sandals (flat or with heels)

Bronze; pewter; nude clutch purse
Dark blue denim jeans
Fitted blazer
Flirty dresses and skirts
Short scarves
Fitted and modern stay at home clothes
Knee length shorts or capris
Detailed tops with visually interesting components

Semi Formal/Formal
Cocktail dress
Formal gown
Glam shoes
Cocktail rings
Dangling earrings

All Segments
Detailed belts (width is important)
Statement earrings and necklaces

A summary of essential staples are as follows:
- Dark/black denim jeans
- White/black fitted button shirt
- Denim shirt
- Cocktail dress in navy/burgundy/pewter/black
- Nude/black pump or sandals
- Pearls (long and short)
- Wrap top or dress
- Statement necklaces or earrings
- Nude/pewter clutch purse
- Black/navy/brown blazer
- Black/navy/brown skirt or pants
- Cocktail ring
- Leather bag in brown/burgundy/black/pewter

" *There is nothing better than knowing that you have a carefully curated wardrobe – both clothes and accessories all ready at the drop of a hat for that impromptu occasion. Sometimes I just open my closet, sit and stare...content in the knowledge that I have several options at my fingertips for work and social events.* "

—JEANETTE B

" *20 pounds overweight and a wardrobe full of size 8 clothes rubbing it in my face, turning 58, professional life, a disaster and my personal life not much better...this was me at the start of 2014. Then I hired Patrice (cheaper than Botox, lipo and a therapist and a far more pleasant experience!). Small things...wearing the right colours and shapes for my skin type and body shape, wearing "statement pieces" of jewelry... in a mere week people were complimenting me on how " fabulous I looked. Great thing though I FELT fabulous. A year later my professional and social lives are back on track. I am still 20 pounds overweight and am now 58, but I look better than I did at 48 and 20 pounds lighter! We owe it to ourselves to be the best of ourselves. Patrice DaCosta helped me to do that!* "

—SHARON C

- Signature scent
- Neutral tone shoes pewter, bronze/black (flats/pumps/ sling back)
- Stylish and functional watch
- Casual cotton or cotton blend dress

Dressing At Home

Moms, wives and women in general, please resist from looking ten years older while you are at home. Your home clothes are just as important, it really shows your true self. Be mindful of your body odor, the state of your hair, underwear and clothes.

This is the perfect time to throw out the torn/ripped dresses/ shirts, avoid wearing baggy pants, unkempt hair, anything that is unattractive. Do not disregard your "home" wardrobe. Remember three things:

- You may have a spouse or partner and social or professional opportunities come when you least expect

- If you are a parent, you should be the best role model to your children

- You do not want your children to be emulating the wrong person(s)

Suggested examples of what to wear at home:

- Leggings/tights with fitted t-shirt or tank top
- Tube top/spaghetti dress (long or short)
- Shorts/camisoles/tank tops
- Track suit or pants
- Avoid large, torn, unattractive clothing

Organize Your Wardrobe and Find Everything You Need Now!

Do you realize your wardrobe is one of the first things you see in the mornings? An unorganized wardrobe can set the tone for your thoughts and your day. My question to you is: What relationship do you have with your wardrobe?

It is best to organize your wardrobe either by colours (e.g. all black, all red) or clothes type (skirt, pants, dresses), Whichever works for you; the important thing is to create a system that works for you and will assist you in looking your best, saving time and being organized.

Your accents are more critical than even your clothes. By accents, I mean, jewelry, scarves, belts, shoes, clutch purses, bags. Create a collection of great accents that can add "oomph" to your wardrobe.

Invest in items conducive for storage and organization. An organized wardrobe is often manifested in an organized look. In addition, you save time and you allow yourself to be more creative as you are able to see what you have, what is needed and what could be. As much as possible, use clear containers and jewelry boxes.

Stoosh suggested items for closet organization

- T-rack for long jewelry
- Hanging jewelry organizer (earrings, brooches, necklaces). These are made in various sizes and types
- Jewelry organizer and mirror combination – a great space saver
- Bracelet holders – two or three levels
- Plastic, slim line or wood hangers, avoid hangars from dry cleaners
- Utensil trays (jewelry and earrings)

- Book ends (clutch purses and bags)
- Ice trays (earrings)
- Clear containers including stackable ones
- Clear shoe boxes, labels
- Over the door shoes, handbag, hat rack
- Zip lock bags

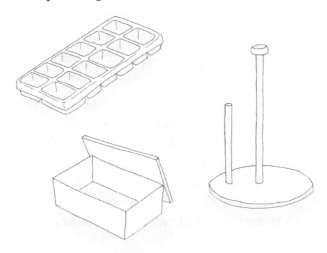

- Nails
- Over the door hooks
- Paper towel holder (vertical ones)
- Large flat bowls

Investing in a closet overhaul is also a great option. After organizing your clothing, it is an amazing idea to redo your closet layout especially if you constantly have clutter or poor usage of space.

Choose the Right Outfit for Every Occasion

I'm often told, "I don't go anywhere so I don't need certain types of clothes". The key is to have a holistic wardrobe and to have something in each category. I am a firm believer that each of us should always have "what-if" days. What if I receive an invitation at a very short notice? What if I get a very great opportunity but was not appropriately attired? What if I am short-changing myself by thinking so limited? Assess yourself before walking through the door. Honesty is best.

If there is an invitation with a dress code, proper etiquette is to comply with what is requested, not what you feel like wearing. If you are not sure, ask your host or dress up so that if needed you can dress down.

Invest in your wardrobe. Mix the various segments (work, church, casual, casually elegant). Do you know your wardrobe is a representation of you? Your likes and dislikes? Your relationship with what's "living" in the wardrobe speaks volume as to your fashion style, how meticulous and detailed you are.

What to Look for in Fabric, Fit and Quality

Choosing fabric

Believe it or not, your choice of fabric factors in more than 60% of your outfit. Poor fabric choice can result in a poor image. Here are a few considerations when choosing fabric for custom or ready-made clothing:

> Weight/structure—how heavy; how thin; your lifestyle— free movement; not much ironing; busy on the go person; your career—executive/formal outfits vs business casual; durability—do I want one wear or longevity? The image you would like to project—successful, progressive image versus cheap look; your body type—do I need to conceal any body part; is the fabric too clingy versus tailored?

Recommended fabrics for clothing are:

- Cotton
- Silk
- Knit
- Polyester blend
- Rayon challis

It is recommended to invest in quality and breathable fabrics. Polyester is one of my least favourite fabrics, as most of my clients know, her name is "Miss Poly". It is a man-made fabric that smells when you perspire and traps heat quite a bit. For those living in tropical climates, please be aware of this fabric. On the plus side, it is great for the very cold bitter days (for those living in colder climates). At times, there is a sheen on the fabric after ironing a few times which is not a very attractive look. Polyester, though durable, should not occupy more than 30% of your wardrobe; aim for a polyester blend. Most companies utilize this fabric for employee uniforms due to durability and cost.

Names of fabrics:

- Tweed
- Wool
- Gingham
- Viscose
- Chiffon
- Corduroy
- Boucle
- Linen
- Hounds tooth
- Paisley

Quality

I cannot emphasize enough the importance of having quality items in your wardrobe. Please note, quality doesn't have to mean expensive. You can find quality pieces on the clearance or mark down racks. Some women believe a closet filled with a lot of items is best versus having items that will last a lifetime. It's the quality not the quantity that matters as you enhance yourself into being "Stoosher". It is best to have 25 great pieces in the wardrobe that can be mixed or matched rather than 100 pieces that are of sub-standard quality; by this I mean, clothing that cannot withstand more than two or three wears without being stretched out or the colour begins to fade. "Cheap clothing isn't cheap"; in the long run it works out to be more expensive. I often encourage my clients to take the time and check the fabric content on the label. Natural fibers such as wool, silk and cotton last longer than synthetics; if cared for correctly.

How do you know a garment is of good quality?

- Stitching and thread – the type of stitches and how much of the thread is visible

- Structure (thin/thick) and type and feel of fabric; is it smooth, rough, hard, soft on the skin?

- Patterns – are normally matched up at the seam, placket, yokes and sleeves

- Details – buttons, pockets, interfacing, double yoke, four buttons instead of three? Any bead work? Are they falling off?

- Seams - the tighter the stitching, the lower the chances of garment being ripped. Are they sewn properly? Pull on both sides of the fabric and see if it pulls apart slightly, if it does, more than likely the garment is not sewn properly

- Thread – colour should match exactly and should be same type as fabric

- Belts – replace self-fabric belt with leather or woven belts. Avoid wearing a plastic belt as this lowers the quality of the outfit

These subtle details will help to identify the quality level of the garment. Please note brand name/designer wear does not always equal quality.

Proper Fit for Standard Clothing

Blouse/Shirt

- Length of blouse should be no shorter than hipbone

- Sleeve length should be at wrist bone

- Sleeve width should be at least 1½ to 1¾ of fabric

- Buttons should remain closed with gaping

- You should have room to move, to bend and stretch your arms

- Skirts

- Underwear should never show

- Skirts should not ride up when you sit. If it passes half of your thigh when you sit chances are it is too short

- Pockets should not gape open

- Waistband should be loose enough to allow for one to two fingers to be inserted, avoid wearing tight skirts at the waist

- Skirts should not curve under buttocks; fabric should lay straight

- Pants/slacks

- Pleats must remain closed
- Panty-line must not show
- Waistband should have no gap or bulge

READY TO WEAR IS NOT ALWAYS POSSIBLE. FINDING A PROPER FIT OFF THE RACK IS SOMETIMES NEXT TO IMPOSSIBLE. IT IS OK TO ALTER A GARMENT ESPECIALLY IF MOST AREAS ARE FITTING WELL. DO NOT PASS UP A GREAT GARMENT BECAUSE OF LITTLE NIPS HERE AND THERE THAT YOU COULD MAKE.

INVEST IN HAVING A HOLISTIC WARDROBE. THE INVESTMENT IS WELL WORTH IT AS YOU WILL EVENTUALLY SPEND LESS.

RESIST FROM BUYING CHEAPLY MADE JEWELRY, BELTS AND HANDBAGS. YOUR ACCESSORIES ARE THE "ICING ON THE CAKE" FOR YOUR APPEARANCE. PAY ATTENTION TO THEM.

Chapter Four

ACCENTUATING YOUR ASSETS AND LESSENING YOUR LIABILITIES

"ANY BODY TYPE IS BEAUTIFUL. IT'S ALL ABOUT LOVING WHAT YOU GOT AND ROCKING IT."

—MEGHAN TRAINOR

Identify Your Body Type

When was the last time you took a very long look at your body? In my experience, I've met so many women who complain about their body; whether it is, a big stomach (the main culprit), large thighs and arms, wide feet, large face, big or small bust, short neck, flat butt or large butt. This list goes on.

We all have assets and liabilities. In other words, we have positives and negatives. The important thing is to identify and enhance our assets but camouflage the liabilities.

What looks like your body type?

The Main Body Types are:
- **Rectangle:** A boyish figure, very little curves, and straight almost like a square.

- **Hourglass:** A defined waist and proportioned butt and hips

- **Pear shaped:** Larger on the bottom than the top
- **Apple shaped:** The challenged area is the stomach, with smaller hips and thighs
- **Inverted triangle:** The shoulder is wider than the hips
- **Triangle:** Hips are wider than shoulder

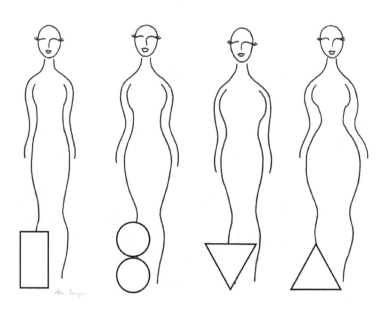

Dress Your Body Type

Not everything you see on a mannequin is for you. You are unique and it's best to try things on, avoid being caught in a fad. Be real with yourself. "Dress for the size you are, not for the size you want to be". By now you should have identified your body type. The question is, how do I look my best at all times?

BALANCING YOUR BODY

CHALLENGE	WHAT TO LOOK FOR
LONG NECKS	HIGH STAND UP COLLARS LONGER HAIRSTYLES
SHORT NECKS	OPEN, V NECKS. SHORTER HAIRSTYLES ANGLED AT THE BACK
SMALL BUST	POCKETS, LAPELS HORIZONTAL DESIGNS LAYERS CREATE ILLUSION OF CURVES
BIG BUST	OPEN/V NECKLINES DROP WAISTLINE IN DRESSES MODERATE SIZE BELTS (SAME COLOUR AS TOP)
BROAD BOTTOM	LONGER JACKETS THAT END BELOW BOTTOM. NO FLAP POCKETS LOOSE WAISTED SKIRTS
HEAVY THIGHS	SOLID/VERTICAL PATTERNS IN PANTS FITTED BUT NOT TIGHT PANTS SOFTLY GATHERED WAISTLINE SKIRTS CULOTTES (COOL-ATS).
THIN LEGS	LONGER SKIRTS LOW OR FLAT HEELS LIGHTER TONE STOCKING
WIDE HIPS	LONGER LINE JACKETS OR SHORTER JACKETS. VERTICAL PATTERNS

Quick Tip

Did You Know Jewelry Can Flatter Your Body Type?

Do not be surprised, wearing jewelry may or may not flatter your body type. Here are a few examples:

1. Rings – The length of your fingers should be in balance with the size of the ring. Long fingers = larger stones and wider ring; short fingers = smaller stones and smaller ring

2. Earrings – The shape of your face is important when choosing an earring. The key is choosing opposites for your face shape.

    a. For a round or circular shaped face, aim for dangling rectangles or square not round studs.

    b. An oval shape can enjoy almost every style.

    c. Square shape should aim for rectangle or circular shapes.

3. Necklace - The shape and size of the necklace, is of utmost importance. Be reminded, the items that are closest to your face, matter the most. Similar to the earrings example, aim for wearing the opposite shapes to your face. When you identify what works for your body and face shape half your battle is won. Note that curvier figures can wear more substantial necklaces.

MANY OF US LOOK AT IMAGES IN MAGAZINES OR TELEVISION AND CANNOT RELATE TO WHAT WE SEE. HOWEVER, WE MUST EMBRACE WHAT WE ARE BLESSED WITH.

Embrace Your Unique Self

Learning about your body is a top priority. For example: The ways to accentuate or camouflage the body, loving your height, your complexion, your hair, your feet, your knees, your hands, your eyes, your lips or your ears. The key to being stylish is knowing your strengths and working with them. Avoid focusing on the negatives.

Many clients have expressed what they believe to be their lack of style and creativity. Comments such as "I have no idea how to match, how to create different looks. I wish I could be as creative as others". Yes there may be some truth that some people are more creative or have a certain stylish edge over others. Even so, we all have some amount of potential in us to bring out our best. Embrace it! If you haven't found it, look for it deep down, it is there.

You will stand out (in a good way). The most frequent excuse I hear from clients, "I want to blend in, I do not want to stand out", and my question is; how do you blend in when you are unique? Whether you want to believe it or not, the minute you walk through the door, you stand out one way or the other – good or bad. Why not aim for the good? As Coco Chanel said, "A stylish woman is one that blends in but stands out at the same time".

Without a doubt, you will feel better about yourself. Why not make your life easier by taking care of how you look. Did you know, how you look has a direct influence on how you feel? Know you are worth the item that looks stunning but cost an extra $25. It is proven that opportunities come more readily when you look the part.

WHAT ARE TWO UNIQUE FEATURES ABOUT YOU? IS IT YOUR HAIR, SMILE, HEIGHT, NOSE, FINGERS, FEET, LEGS, EYES? WHATEVER IT IS, TAKE A MINUTE TO IDENTIFY.

Stoosh Advice

- Not sure what to buy when shopping? Follow the most stylish person in the store. Look at what he/she is looking at or buying.

- It is important to get your body type analyzed so you can know what styles are flattering and those that are not.

- Stop settling for unnecessary bargains. It is not a bargain if it is hanging in your closet unworn.

Dress nicely when shopping. You will have a "pep" in your step and choosing an outfit will be more fulfilling. In addition, people speak to you based on what they see. The sales associates will treat and speak to you differently. Guaranteed!

Build your wardrobe based on your own objectives, and not your friends'. If you are tired of having a blah wardrobe and your aim is to add some creativity and an out-of-the-box experience, do not allow your friend, who is on a different level, to influence your choices and you purchase the same-old-same-old. At the end of the day you only get upset with yourself and nothing changes. However, if your friend is stylish and creative, that's a good person to tag along with on your next shopping trip.

Chapter Five

ACCESSORIZE YOUR PROFESSIONAL & LEISURE WARDROBE

"ANY OPPORTUNITY TO ADORN ONESELF IS HUMAN, AND ACCESSORIES ARE AN EASY WAY TO DO IT."—MARC JACOBS

Do you know accessories should be 25% of your wardrobe budget? Accessories are the "icing on the cake" for an outfit. It makes no sense to have accessories that are not working for you. Avoid purchasing accessories only because of price. I often hear the lament, "it was on sale, so I bought it". Many times that piece becomes a dust collector as it is not worn. Accessories can enhance your outfits.

The right accessories can also add or take away from your first impression. Investing in enough pieces can help to save money. Do not be surprised, accessories extend the versatility of an outfit allowing more than one look.

Avoid making excuses, find the accessories that are right for you.

The key is to have a mixture of accessories. Refrain from limiting yourself to one type of jewelry. Some clients only wear costume or real metal or leather in everything. A variety of styles allow for more creativity.

Must Have Accessories

- Brooches: every shape and colour
- Belts with great focal point and colours
- Quality handbag/s with interesting hardware
- Scarves (small/medium size) in your complimentary colours: to tie on bags/around the neck which adds a pop of colour, used as a belt
- Cocktail rings with interesting details
- Neutral tone shoes (flats/heels/sling back) nude, pewter, and bronze, black, burgundy
- Pearls (short and long) in all colours
- Unusual necklaces
- Gold/diamond earring or necklace

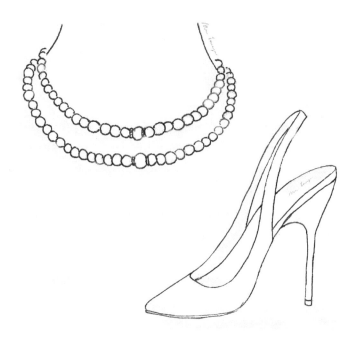

Keep Proportion and Quality in Mind

In real estate, the adage is: Location, Location, Location. In fashion, it's Proportion, Proportion, Proportion. I cannot stress the importance. The size of your accessories are guided by your height, five feet, four inches and under is considered petite (please note petite is not by weight but height), these individuals should aim for small accessories and small prints in fabrics. An average height is five feet, five inches to five feet, seven inches, small to medium sizes are more appropriate. Taller individuals wear medium to large scale accessories and print.

A two-inch belt is a standard size for most body types. The important thing is to ensure nothing overpowers you when placed on your body (whether a belt, handbag, jewelry or colour). A belt is too large when it covers half of your torso which in return gives the perception that you are shorter or fuller than you are. If your torso is long, you can go slightly wider as long as your height and body type allow it.

Your handbag is too large if it is the first thing that is seen before your face. Another quick trick is, to place handbag between your waist and knee if the bag takes up more than half of your thigh chances are it is too big.

High quality is important in all areas of your style, but even more for accessories. Quality doesn't have to be overwhelmingly pricey. You can have accessories that are not necessarily expensive but have style. However, a good handbag is key to a female's look, if I am asked what a good accessory splurge is, my answer would be the handbag/pocketbook. It says a lot about how detailed, fashionable, and meticulous you are. The equivalent splurge for a male is quality shoes or male bag.

When examining the quality of accessories, some key areas to look for are:

- **The stitching** – is it concealed or outside, look at the finish. Is it messy or well done? Does the item look cheap or of high quality? Stitching is vitally important on items such as shoes, handbags, wallets, clutch purses and belts.

- **The clasp, placement of stones** – especially important for brooches, necklaces, bracelets, hair accessories, earrings.

- **Material and fabric** – leather versus non leather can make a difference with belts, handbags, wallets, clutch purses and shoes. Tie fabric—silk versus polyester. Cotton socks versus cotton blend.

Other accessories (some might surprise you):

Necklaces, earrings, bracelets, rings, shoes, handbags, brooches, belts, scarves, hair accessories, sunglasses, prescription glasses, stockings, socks, ties, tie pins, wallets, clutch purses, messenger bags, hats/caps, fascinators, handkerchief.

How to Store Your Accessories

- Ice trays, egg tray
- Utensil trays, clear shoe box
- Hanging clear pockets, stackable trays
- Scarf or belt hangar
- Small to medium sized bowls (glass/wood/ceramic)
- Handbag holder, cap holder
- Hat boxes, bracelet holder
- Divider shelves

- Hangars, saucers,

- Paper towel holder (vertical ones)

- Over the door or under the bed shoe holders

- Cardboard sheet from Christmas pepper lights

- Socks/draw partitions

- Shadow boxes

- Muffin tins

- Jewelry tree

- Storage bins

- Jewelry neck stands

ACCESSORIES ON AN OUTFIT IS LIKE MAKEUP ON THE FACE. IT ADDS THE RIGHT FINISHING TOUCH

ORGANIZED ACCESSORIES = SAVED TIME = ORGANIZED LOOKS

AVOID PLACING YOUR JEWELRY IN A DRAWER WITHOUT SECTIONS/PARTITIONS. THAT IS CHAOS

Chapter Six

HOW TO BE STOOSH (CREATING GOOD FIRST IMPRESSIONS)

"WITH ME IT'S ALWAYS ABOUT FIRST IMPRESSIONS."—BILLY ZANE

The Stoosh Woman at Work and Play

Stoosh: Stylish, sophisticated and successful; think about those words. Which word best describes you? One, two, all or none? Whatever you thought of, the important thing is to give yourself permission to get to the next level.

A Stoosh woman is one who wears clothes that expresses her lifestyle and personality; is modern but classic and knows how to blend both; appreciates her body type and knows how to dress appropriately; not afraid to wear quality clothing to enhance her assets; knows what is appropriate for the occasion; possesses a versatile wardrobe that allows her to express her personality in a creative and stylish manner and certainly not afraid to mix modern with classic.

She is also aware of the importance of a good image and the impact it has on her reputation. Knowing her colours is also essential, she knows the impact of wearing the right shade versus buying anything just because. The Stoosh woman takes care of her body, not just her image, going to the spa, getting a manicure and

"*Being a "Stoosh" professional woman provides me with such a sense of freedom! On a daily basis it also gives me a real foundation of confidence. Having a series of coordinated outfits put together to suit the mental image of the person I want to project is very, very liberating. Knowing each combination enhances my best features and looks good and well thought out is a treasure indeed…and the regular compliments and positive comments on my appearance don't hurt either.*

Having the outfit combinations pre-planned by Patrice also removes stress and aids in speedy dressing in the mornings. For those of us who travel a lot, whether on business or pleasure, it is a blessing to have pictures of the ensemble combinations, so that when packing everything is remembered, from jewelry, handbags, shoes, etc. Finally…no more arriving somewhere and realizing you left the necklace, belt, bag or scarf that really finishes that otherwise fabulous look which turns heads and says "wow".

The best part is knowing that everything in my wardrobe is there for a reason or occasion, and when I do go shopping being able to maximize the impact of my new purchases. There is also the thrill of regularly going shopping in my own wardrobe and creating new outfits myself based on pieces that I might have had for years. To be a "Stoosh" woman is to look "Superlative" all the time! Thanks Patrice. "

—BRENDA P

pedicure frequently as well as regular hair appointments are all important. She enjoys sharing with others and giving to the less fortunate.

At play, she enjoys a good laugh, enjoys having good friends around and entertains when necessary. Her casual looks are visually interesting with attention to details. Her humility and confidence is often seen by many. Her fashion style can be classic, dramatic, creative, sporty or feminine. She is not afraid to make changes and to improve. Her confidence and liberation has allowed her to be free both from the inside and out. What others say matters very little as she knows what works and doesn't for her.

At work, she is highly professional and ensures her attire speaks volume. Attending corporate events is high on the list.

The Stoosh Man at Work and Play

The Stoosh man, yes many do exist. Some men tend to think being groomed or focusing on image is not masculine enough. He is stylish, certainly not afraid to experiment in mixing colours and prints. Usually, he's metrosexual (a heterosexual, urban man who enjoys shopping, fashion, and similar interests). He's trendy and owns a versatile wardrobe. He invests wisely in his outfits and accessories are often not compromised. Don't be surprised if his wardrobe is strategically laid out and he owns a lot of clothes. The aim is to have the correct pieces so whether at work or play he will portray a good image.

The Stoosh man is poised and sociable and fun to be around. He buys from specific stores and builds up a relationship with them to ensure he gets the best offers and good service.

At play, he is casual but again, simple details are often noticed in his shirt, belt, or shorts even a mere jeans pants. Proper fit is high on the list, he also knows the importance of having a good tailor to ensure alterations can be made.

At work, his work wardrobe speaks volumes. A high level of confidence and professionalism is often exhibited. Appropriately garbed at corporate events and entertaining clients are standard. The Stoosh man who owns his business is not afraid to entertain clients and give quality gifts.

Can an Organization be Stoosh? Yes!

The Stoosh Company is a Poised, Professional Workforce.

Expressing Your Unique Style in Uniforms

Uniforms are often used as a camouflage by many employees, but one of the most important features is that it represents a corporate entity's brand. When wearing uniforms, extra attention must be made. Details will play a vital role in ensuring your uniforms are worn correctly and represent your company's image. Enhancing your uniform with details and accessories is a good idea. However, be mindful that not because something is in fashion means it is appropriate for work. The operative word is *Professionalism.*

Details to consider are:

1. Hairstyle – ensure the colour and style of your hair are appropriate for work. Example: Wearing purple and multi-colour hued hair.

2. Accessories – ensure that your accessories enhance rather than detract from your uniform. Example: Wearing punk rock accessories to a corporate uniform.

3. Makeup – ensure makeup is not outlandish.

Professionalism at events—holiday parties, dinners and ceremonies

Apart from dressing appropriately at company sponsored events, it's important to behave appropriately. Be mindful there is a Monday after attending that staff party or corporate event; be mindful of your behavior, your attire and conduct. Technology makes everything easily accessible—your wild dance could be someone's status update on social media the morning after.

Here are some **do's** and **don't's**:

DO

- Make a point of speaking with people who you don't usually get a chance to speak with in the organization
- Show interest in their lives without prying e.g. travel, children, hobbies
- Be polite and courteous to all
- Know basic dining etiquette – which fork goes with what etc.
- Shake hands firmly and maintain eye contact
- Mingle
- Upgrade your work clothes for the event
- Upgrade your accessories for the event.

DON'T

- Have more than one or two drinks
- Cultivate intimate relationships
- Use bad language
- Dance suggestively

- Over talk or monopolize the conversation
- Under talk or be a wallflower
- Be loud
- Eat while talking
- Talk about politics or religion
- Dress as if going to a night club
- Show too much skin or body parts
- Wear tight, slinky or suggestive clothing.

Chapter Seven

YOU WEAR WHAT FOR BUSINESS CASUAL?

"I USED TO WORK FOR A MANAGEMENT CONSULTING COMPANY, SO I DRESSED DIFFERENTLY— BUSINESS CASUAL, PROBABLY A LOT OF THINGS FROM BANANA REPUBLIC. MY WARDROBE NOW IS DEFINITELY MORE EXPENSIVE, BUT I ALWAYS DRESS FOR THE OCCASION."

—JOHN LEGEND

Business casual—when I hear this word I often cringe. My experience as a personal development expert allows me the opportunity to interact with corporations in various sectors. Many companies are having a challenging time as employees are forgetting the word that comes before casual...***Business!***

Business casual is a more relaxed but professional look that is often mistaken for being too relaxed. It is the middle-ground between business and street wear. Your attire should be clean, unwrinkled and ready to wear to an impromptu meeting or to meet a client. Appropriate business casual sets the tone for opportunities. Do not confuse business casual with picnic or night club attire.

If your industry is more relaxed, in its dressing, that's no excuse to wear inappropriate clothing to the office. Professionalism is key to the success of wearing business casual. You enter the door of a corporation to conduct business, so look the part.

Even though a certain type of style may be in fashion, that doesn't mean it is appropriate for the workplace. For example: Skinny fit or tight pants; very short and tight skirts and fluorescent colours. Aim for classic rather than trendy.

Three considerations for business casual:
1. Attention to detail:
Little things can have a huge impact. Details can have both negative and positive effect on your personal presentation. Keep accessories simple and neat. Placement and conditions of buttons; zippers are closed and functioning; ensuring your shoes are clean, appropriate and comfortable for the workplace.

2. Fit of clothing:
You represent the company even on casual days. It is important to avoid tight or too big clothing. Both women and men should realize tight clothing in particular does not create a good first impression. I am often asked what is considered tight clothing. Tight is when there are gaps in pockets; buttons, the clothing is pulling, it is difficult to breathe, or you can't sit; clothes pinch you, skirt or pants ride up several inches.

3. Quality of clothing:
Quality is better than quantity. Invest in a few key pieces that will last a lifetime especially if your career lends for this type of clothing. Look at it as investing in your personal brand. On a casual day you might be called to attend a meeting and represent your company or yourself if you're self-employed.

What to Wear

- Khakis, corduroy, twill, cotton pants
- Wrap and sheath dresses
- Fitted long sleeve cotton shirts
- Polo or short sleeve shirts with collar
- Pencil or straight skirts
- Flats/loafers/sling back shoes
- Leather belt
- Cardigans/twin sets
- Blazer
- Classic accessories (pearls, silver, gold, semi-precious stones)
- Dark denim
- Brooches

What Not to Wear

- Graphic t-shirts
- Ripped/broken belt
- Very strappy open toe sandals
- Light wash denim; denim with sequins and rips
- Sneakers
- Flip flops
- Linen
- Sweatshirts
- Shorts/crop tops
- Baseball hats and bandanas

- Nail polish in neon colours and extravagant designs
- Oversized jewelry
- Zippered hoodie
- Spaghetti straps
- Strongly scented cologne or perfume
- Low-rise pants that when viewed from behind, show the butterfly tattoo or the "crack" when you sit.

BEFORE MAKING A CAREER CLOTHING PURCHASE, ASK YOURSELF THE FOLLOWING: CAN I WEAR THIS TO AN IMPROMPTU MEETING? WOULD I BE DRESSED APPROPRIATELY IF A CLIENT SHOULD SEE ME? WHAT THREE WAYS CAN I WEAR THIS AND WHAT THREE PLACES CAN IT BE WORN?

BUSINESS CASUAL SHOULD NOT BE A FAD (TEMPORARY); CLASSIC AND TIMELESS ITEMS ARE RECOMMENDED.

Chapter Eight

PUTTING YOUR BEST FACE FORWARD WHEREVER YOU ARE

*"I'M A BIG BELIEVER IN THAT
IF YOU FOCUS ON GOOD SKIN CARE,
YOU REALLY WON'T NEED
A LOT OF MAKEUP."*—DEMI MOORE

The skin, so often overlooked, is such an important part of our bodies, our lives and is part of our communication center. The condition of your skin can be influenced by hereditary factors but very often it's impacted by lifestyle choices:

What are you eating?

Are you getting enough sleep?

Are you drinking enough water?

Are you using the right products for your skin type?

How much exercise are you doing?

Do you smoke?

Do you replenish your skin with much needed moisture?

Too much sun exposure?

Many women disregard their skin. When asked what skin care regime you have, I often hear "not much, I don't have the time or I can't be bothered".

This is your skin, you have to and need to take charge. When was the last time you evaluated your face, the condition, the texture of your skin? We are guilty of going through the door without moisture, without sunscreen, without any form of protection as we face the elements whether it is sun, snow or rain; our skin calls for some type of shield. Unprotected skin can cause brown spots, premature wrinkling, and poor skin texture.

One of my favourite makeup artists, Bobbi Brown, suggests the following Skin Care Necessities that I agree is good to incorporate in any beauty regimen:

- Gel cleanser: gentle, non-stripping formula for oily skin. In hot weather use for all skin types
- Non oily makeup remover
- Eye cream
- Body lotion and oil
- Pumice stone: smooth rough spots and calluses on feet

Identify Your Skin Type

There are four main skin types:

1. Normal

This is the skin type that is envied among women and men. This skin type is next to perfection. Normal skin is not too dry, not too oily and has the following characteristics:

- None or few imperfections
- No severe sensitivity
- Barely visible pores
- A radiant complexion

2. Combination

As the name suggests, it is a culmination of two skin types: dry or normal in some areas and oily in others, such as the T-zone (nose, forehead, and chin). Many people have combination skin, which may benefit from slightly different types of skin care in different areas. Combination skin is prone to blackheads, shiny skin, and large pores.

3. Dry Skin

When exposed to drying factors the skin can crack, peel, or become itchy, irritated, or inflamed. If your skin is very dry, it can become rough and scaly, especially on the back of your hands, arms, and legs.

The usual characteristics of dry skin are:

- Almost invisible pores
- Dull, rough complexion
- Red patches
- Less elasticity
- More visible lines

4. Oily Skin

- Enlarged pores
- Dull or shiny, thick complexion
- Blackheads, pimples, or other blemishes

SOURCE: WWW.WEBMD.COM

A fifth type of skin is the sensitive skin. This type of skin is prone to itchiness, rashes and redness. Care must be taken in selecting the right non-allergenic products or avoid foods and environmental factors that may trigger this condition.

Skincare for the tropics

A few common misconceptions are associated with being in the tropics. The first is that moisturizer is not needed due to the abundance of sweat. Why add more moisture to the skin when the skin is already "moisturized" naturally? The answer is that we need to replenish the skin so it remains supple and smooth.

Another misconception is that sun block is only for Caucasians and very fair-skinned people. Many individuals (male and female) fail to realize that even a minute of exposure can start the process of sun damage. Granted, darker skin has more melanin but care must still be taken to protect the skin with a wide-brimmed hat, sun glasses for the delicate eye area and sunscreen.

Cleansing the Skin

I recently discovered, cleansing doesn't have to be with an actual product. Water by itself, especially in the mornings, especially for those with larger pores, does the trick.

Using your cleanser nightly is good enough. It took me some time to adjust but I can certainly see the difference with my pores. I have to credit my aesthetician, Krystl, who made the suggestion. The important thing is to ensure that your face is clean. Of course, to remove your make-up you would use cleanser or make up removal pads.

When cleansing, ensure you gently dab your face, not in a forceful pull-down manner. Your skin is delicate.

Moisturizing the Skin

Any organ needs moisture to function at its optimum; the skin is no different. The key to adding moisture to the skin is the amount applied. Too much is often applied which results in an oily or greasy appearance. When applying your moisturizer, always use upward movements instead of downward. This is especially helpful as we get older.

Exfoliating the Skin

Exfoliate the skin once or twice per week and depending on the product, once every two weeks. Some products are harsher than others. Exfoliating the body at least twice a month is great for renewing your skin.

Skincare for Cooler Climates

Winter can be harsh on the skin resulting in cracking, itching and flaky, dry skin. Before travelling to cooler climes, here are a few tips to consider:

- Hydrate your body

  To maintain beautiful skin, drink lots of water. It's really true that beautiful skin starts from the inside out. Whenever you are on the go, always carry a bottle of water. Add a spritz of lemon for a different taste from plain water. You will also achieve a healthy glow.

- Wear sunscreen

  Yes, even in winter you need sunscreen. The sun's rays can still damage your skin. Always protect your skin from the sun's aging tendency.

- Replenish your skin with moisturizer

  I cannot emphasize moisturizing your skin enough! The moisturizer you use in summer should be switched to a more appropriate (or heavier) one for winter. Avoid using baby oil and body oil as the mineral contents in them can clog your pores.

- Eat healthy foods

  While on the road, we have a tendency to eat anything that's available. Consciously select foods that will nourish your skin and body: Omega-rich foods; nuts; as well as fruits and vegetables that are packed with Vitamin C. Note that Vitamin C is essential for collagen stimulation and aids in cell renewal.

- Protect your lips

  Your lips tend to quickly get dry and chapped during the winter months. Indoor heat does not help. Use a nurturing lip balm, like Blistex to restore your lips to softness.

- Pay attention to your hands and feet

  The skin on your hands and feet has fewer oil glands than the rest of your body. It's always exposed to the elements so cracking and itching can develop. You want to give your skin some TLC by:

  - Moisturizing your hands with coconut oil mixed with Vitamin E oil and wearing a glove to bed at night

  - Do the same for your feet and wear socks to bed.

  - Keep your hands and feet supple during the day with extra-moisturizing lotions

  - Get regular pedicures even though you are not wearing sandals. A good pedicure at a salon will ensure that the dead skin cells are exfoliated

Take showers instead of baths

Even though it may feel welcoming after a cold day, a long, hot bath can actually dry out your skin. Use warm not hot water for your shower.

Skincare for Warmer Climates

- Avoid using heavy lotion on your skin. Mixed with sweat, it can clog your pores

- Use a light weight moisturizer and don't forget to apply

sunscreen. Select a broad-spectrum sunscreen between SPF 30 and 50. Using a higher SPF can be harmful to your skin. Moisturizers with SPF 15 is not much sun protection

- Dress in light fabrics so your skin can breathe and not get overheated. Cotton and linen are good bets. Also wear light colours to deflect the heat from your body rather than dark colours which absorb heat

- Drink lots of water. As your body loses water from sweating under the hot sun, you will need to replenish by hydrating your body

Three Minute Face: Minimum Makeup

- Apply foundation to make skin look flawless

- Use concealer under the eyes and in the most recessed corners of the eyes. It diminishes dark shadows and makes you look more awake

- Try a tinted moisturizer or, if your skin is smooth naturally, sweep a natural blush colour or bronzer on your cheeks.

- Apply black or brown mascara

- Finish off your three minute face by applying sheer or lightly tinted lip gloss

The Five Minute Face: Day Makeup

- Apply foundation to even out your skin for a flawless look. Blend carefully

- Apply concealer, focusing on the inner corners of your eyes

- Set concealer and foundation using a brush or puff

- Use a brush to dust highlighter all over the lid, from the lash line to the eyebrow
- Line the eye, using darkest shadow
- Apply one to two coats of black or brown mascara
- Brush blush on the apple of cheeks
- Apply lipstick

FOR EXTRA SKIN HYDRATION MIX BODY OIL WITH LOTION.

HOME REMEDIES:

- CORNMEAL AND BANANA (SOFTEN FEET); HONEY AND CORNMEAL (FACE MASK) OLIVE OIL AND COCONUT OIL ARE GREAT FOR HANDS AND FEET (ESPECIALLY NIGHT TIME)

- TO EXFOLIATE LIPS USE A TOOTHBRUSH ON YOUR LIPS TO REMOVE DEAD CELLS. LIPS WILL FEEL LIKE NEW

- HIGHLIGHT EYEBROWS WITH WHITE EYE PENCIL TO GIVE THE ILLUSION OF A MORE "OPEN" EYE

SOME MEN OFTEN THINK THEIR SKIN IS SO TOUGH THAT SKIN CARE IS NOT AS IMPORTANT. IT IS SUCH A JOY TO SEE MEN REALIZE THAT IS FAR FROM THE TRUTH. THE SUN DOESN'T KNOW YOUR SKIN BELONGS TO A MALE OR FEMALE, IT BURNS JUST THE SAME. SUNSCREEN, CLEANSING, MOISTURIZING, EXFOLIATING AND FACIALS ARE SOME OF THE RECOMMENDED WAYS TO ENSURE A HEALTHY SKIN.

Chapter Nine

TRAVELLING STOOSH STYLE

"I WANT MY HANDBAGS AND MY SHOES TO BE STYLISH BUT I WANT TO MAKE SURE THAT THEY'RE VERSATILE. I TRAVEL AND I HAVE TO MAKE SURE THE PIECES I PUT INTO MY BAG CAN GO WITH A DRESS OR WITH SHORTS OR JEANS."—MARIA SHARAPOVA

If you travel regularly, it is imperative to look stylish while on the go. Please do not disregard your look while at the airport, on the plane, train, bus or in your car. You never know when an opportunity will arise, or who you'll meet. It is also proven that some airlines do upgrade your seating class based on your dress.

One of the main considerations for travel is the fabric of choice which is dependent on your destination weather.

Cardigans/blazers are great to travel with as they can dress up a basic outfit. They keep you warm in airports and chilly airplanes.

Suggested travel outfits are:

- Dark denim/long sleeve button down or plain shirt/blazer with heels or nice flats

- Comfortable slacks with detailed top/cardigan/blazer

- Dress (rayon/jersey) with cardigan, beaded sandals

- Knee length shorts/camisole/blazer or dark denim jacket/ wedges or flats

- Structured leggings/ long tunic top/ scarf and pumps or flats

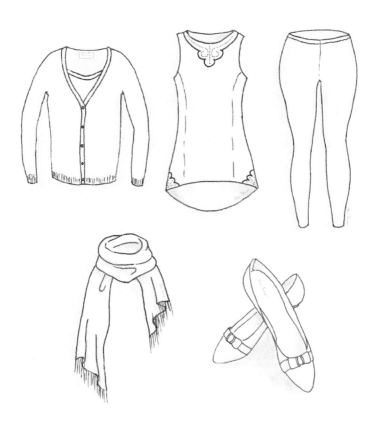

Essential Items to Pack for Women and Men

- Sunscreen, skin care products, hand and body lotion
- Comfortable shoes, sandals
- Blazer, cardigan, shawl
- Accessories that can be worn with more than one outfit (silver, gold, black, burgundy, olive green)
- Dark denim or black jeans
- Slacks and button down shirts
- White fitted shirt
- Plastic bags for wet or dirty clothes
- Vitamins
- Your favourite electronic gadget or book
- Stylish tote or messenger bag
- Sunglasses

Men

- Swim trunks
- Flip flop/shoes
- Shorts/pants
- Casual and dress shirt
- Sunshades
- Exercise gear

  NB:*The focus should be on the fabric to facilitate the weather*

What to Pack for Cooler Climes

- Trench coat
- Winter coat
- Sweaters/cardigans
- Camisoles/vests
- Leggings/tights
- Pants in corduroy/denim/velvet
- Scarves/gloves
- Socks
- Closed shoes (flats/heels), sneaker shoe
- Beret or hat with sequins or brooch
- Rechargeable batteries and chargers

What to Pack for Warmer Climes

- Sundresses
- Swimsuit/cover up
- Cotton dresses and blouses
- Sandals/water shoes
- Shawl/cardigan
- Socks
- Camera
- Zip lock bags/plastic bags
- Guidebook/map
- Personal grooming kit
- Undergarments

- Accessories (jewelry/belt)
- Messenger bag
- Sunglasses
- Sunscreen

Packing for a Caribbean Cruise

- Stylish cover ups to add pizazz to your bathing suit
- Medium sized straw bag
- Beaded sandals for day and evening
- Cotton tube or spaghetti dresses
- Bathing suits (at least three which flatter the body)
- Sunscreen SPF 45 or higher
- Flip flops for the beach or pool
- Water shoes
- Casually elegant tops and dresses
- Motion sickness tabs or wrist bands
- Umbrella
- Shorts
- Shawls/shrugs/pashminas/cardigans
- Hair accessories for bad hair days (hair pins/hair clips)
- A good book and great music
- Sunglasses
- Exercise gear
- Flats and wedge shoes
- Dark wash jeans or black

- Bronze, pewter or camel clutch
- Travel size shampoo/conditioner
- Full size body and facial moisturizer
- Tooth brush/toothpaste
- Razor
- Mini nail polish
- Rechargeable batteries and chargers
- Accessories

Packing for a Mediterranean Cruise

- Cardigans /shawls/scarves
- Sewing kit (emergencies)
- Sandals/walking shoes/flip flops
- Undergarment
- Toiletries
- Camera
- Euros
- Personal grooming products
- Shorts
- Jacket
- Cover up
- Bathing suit
- Sundresses
- Casually elegant dresses, tops and bottoms
- Dressy pants suit

- Lightweight clothing for layering (cover up for religious buildings)
- Blazer/tie (men)
- Flat shoes and elegant ones
- Bronze, pewter, camel clutch
- Opaque tights or leggings
- Travel size umbrella

ALWAYS PACK A COMPLETE OUTFIT (UNDERWEAR/ CLOTHES), MEDICINES IN YOUR HAND LUGGAGE; IN THE EVENT CHECKED BAGS GET LOST OR LEFT BEHIND BY THE AIRLINE.

NEVER TRAVEL WITHOUT A SHAWL/CARDIGAN OR BLAZER AS AIRPORTS AND AIRCRAFT ARE ALWAYS CHILLY.

AVOID WEARING FLIP FLOPS OR BEING TOO CASUAL WHEN TRAVELING. AIM FOR CASUALLY-ELEGANT.

Chapter Ten

IT'S A WRAP!

Putting it all Together—
A Polished Professional You!

As we wrap things up, remember you are your best brand. You are branded wherever you go especially if you represent a corporate entity; even on weekends you are associated with that corporation. Your appearance is your visual resume. Ensure you leave "brand equity" in the form of positive impressions.

People speak to you based on what they see.

What are they seeing?

Always remember you are in charge of your own brand, no one else is. See yourself the way you want to be seen and take the necessary steps to make that change.

My suggested change formula is:

Visualize

How do you see yourself? Is there someone you aspire to be? Align yourself with a "lion" or mentor that you can draw knowledge and inspiration from, whether in your industry or someone you can relate to. It's OK to day dream and see yourself in the future.

Do you know that your thinking dictates your behavior?

Affirm

There is power in the spoken word. Be mindful of what you say. Your words will come to life before you know it. What you proclaim to or about yourself often comes to reality.

What kind of affirmations are you putting into your space?

Act

What action do you need to take to become a better you? What first step do you need to take? Just make the move. Stop procrastinating. Always remember you are worth every sacrifice or investment.

It's often said, small things can become big things. Details are considered the icing on the cake for your personal development. Whether it is your facial expression, hair, teeth, nails, body language, shoes, overall hygiene, your clothes, taking that extra minute can make all the difference in the outcome of your message. You deserve that extra minute or two, please do not feel guilty.

Final Checklist:

☑ Ensure your visual (appearance/facial expression), vocal (your tone) and verbal (what you say) are always sending positive signals

☑ When traveling, please remember you are interfacing with many people, you never know who you will meet. Dress and act the part

☑ Love what you have. We are all unique and wonderfully made. Ensure you focus on ways to enhance and not detract. Look in the mirror, what are the awesome things about you? Say them out loud

☑ Keep a pleasant demeanor, what you give out you often get back

☑ Stop Stressing and Start Living. Dress your body for the size you are not the size you want to be.

☑ Your "**YOU**" asset is all you've got

☑ **Maximize your potential!**

STOOSH
FAVES & RESOURCES

Accessories: Jewelry/Handbags

Jan's Accent – Jamaica

Reve Jewelry - Jamaica

Avark – Barbados

Earth's Jewelry – New York

Clothing

Heather Laine – Jamaica

Bill Edwards – Jamaica

Klutch Boutique – New York

Lord & Taylor Department Store

Martindales – Barbados

Spa

Krysbell Spa - Barbados

Jencare Skin Farm – New York and Jamaica

Soothing Touch Spa – Barbados

Beauty Salon

The Salon – Kingston, Jamaica

Dejavu – Barbados

Jonothan Elliott - Barbados

ABOUT THE AUTHOR

Patrice DaCosta works with both private and corporate clients in the areas of color analysis, wardrobe and style analysis, personal shopping, wardrobe evaluation and makeover, etiquette and personal development. As CEO of Stoosh Images since 2005, she focuses on a holistic approach to style and beauty, combining the outer image that we portray to others, in tandem with developing the inner image of ourselves.

Trained by Dominique Isbecque, Internationally renowned Image Consultant at the Image Resource Center in NY, Patrice is committed to the image industry. She earned a Professional Diploma in Fashion Merchandising from the Professional Career Development Institute in Atlanta. She is also a graduate of the Barbizon School of Modeling, New York.

Patrice earned a Master of Science at the University of Salford, Manchester, England. She also holds a Bachelor of Science degree from the University of Technology, Kingston, Jamaica.

Patrice believes in giving back to the community, as a result, Stoosh Images is affiliated with the following charitable organizations:

- Dress for Success Professional Women's Group
- Save Foundation, Barbados
- Various Childrens' Orphanages in Jamaica

Based in New York City, Patrice serves the entire Caribbean Diaspora and may be contacted at patrice@stooshimages.com

STOOSH GIFT CERTIFICATES

BRIGHTEN SOMEONE'S DAY!

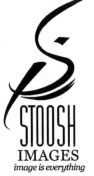

Give the gift that's bound to fit and please your recipient. A Stoosh Gift of Style Certificate makes a great employee incentive that will be appreciated. It is also perfect for graduations, the holidays, wedding showers, birthdays and just because you care.

Gift Certificates are available for any service in increments of $50.00

Select from any service:

- Wardrobe evaluation and makeover
- Colour sessions
- Shopping trips
- Wellness retreats

- Individual consultation
- Communication coaching
- Special events styling

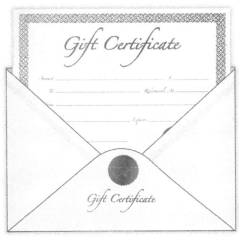

Show your love and regard by reserving your gift certificate today:
patrice@stooshimages.com   www.stooshimages.com